A Practical Guide for New Parents

by

Benjamin D. Gordon, M.D.

DORRANCE PUBLISHING CO
EST. 1920
PITTSBURGH, PENNSYLVANIA 15238

The contents of this work, including, but not limited to, the accuracy of events, people, and places depicted; opinions expressed; permission to use previously published materials included; and any advice given or actions advocated are solely the responsibility of the author, who assumes all liability for said work and indemnifies the publisher against any claims stemming from publication of the work.

All Rights Reserved
Copyright © 2019 by Benjamin D. Gordon, M.D.

No part of this book may be reproduced or transmitted, downloaded, distributed, reverse engineered, or stored in or introduced into any information storage and retrieval system, in any form or by any means, including photocopying and recording, whether electronic or mechanical, now known or hereinafter invented without permission in writing from the publisher.

Dorrance Publishing Co
585 Alpha Drive
Pittsburgh, PA 15238
Visit our website at *www.dorrancebookstore.com*

ISBN: 978-1-4809-9475-1
eISBN: 978-1-4809-9432-4

*Dedicated to the parents who have just
Had their first baby
In the hope that they will realize
That caring for a new baby
Has been done many, many times
And they can do it too
Just as well as anyone else
And—
Maybe better*

CONTENTS

PREFACE vii
1. Formula Making Simplified 1
2. Feeding --- The Traps That Cause Trouble 5
3. Breast Feeding 9
4. Pacifiers and Thumb Sucking 13
5. Sleep – How To Get It When You Want It 17
6. Solids – What, When and Why 21
7. Water 23
8. Skin Care 25
9. Elimination 29
10. Sneezes, Stuffiness and Hiccups 31
11. Outdoors and Indoors 33
12. Toilet Training or Better Still "Learning Control" 35
13. Safety Points and Some Comments
    on "Friendly Advice" 39

14. Some General Points About Sickness
    and What You Should Know About Fever 41
15. How To Give Nose Drops Properly
    for Nasal Problems and To Relieve Earache 45
16. Vomiting and Diarrhea- How To Control Most Cases
    Using Clear Liquids and Careful Feeding 49
17. Avoiding Eating Problems 53
18. Some Points About Growth and Development 57
19. Discipline 59

PREFACE

This volume is a compilation of facts and explanations which my patients have found useful in the care of their new babies.

The aim of this book is to provide new parents with an idea of how normal infants may differ. By understanding this, they can save themselves a lot of unnecessary worry. Expecting a baby to do only certain things, or trying to force the infant into a routine, will surely make the whole family tense and frustrated. For example, every woman knows she will feel weepy and odd for two to four weeks after delivery. This doesn't prevent her from feeling that way but it does help her handle it. She understands it's natural and nothing is wrong. In the same way, the information in these pages will not prevent all problems in babies but it will make them easier to handle.

CHAPTER 1

A SIMPLIFIED WAY TO MAKE FORMULA

New mothers seem to be worried about making formula. The following technique takes less time, is flexible, and can help save money.

1.) Wash bottles and nipples in warm, soapy water, using bottle and nipple brushes to reach all corners.

2.) Force soapy water and then rinse water through each nipple to be sure opening is not clogged.

3.) Rinse bottles and nipples thoroughly in clear, warm water.

4.) Fill each bottle with water *directly from the tap* and put the nipple and cap in place.

5.) Make sure each cap is *loose* before putting the bottles up to boil.

6.) Add water to the sterilizer so that the level is just below the level of the fluid inside the bottles.

7.) Begin timing after the water in the sterilizer has begun to boil and let it boil for twenty-five minutes.

8.) After twenty-five minutes, take the bottles out and let them stand at room temperature. When they're cool, tighten the caps. There is no need to refrigerate them since they just have water in them.

9.) To feed your baby, simply take a bottle of water, add the prescribed number of scoops (each can has a scoop which is usually a tablespoon measure), shake, and feed.

There is no need to heat the bottle since it is not cold and did not come out of the refrigerator. If liquid formula is preferred this can of liquid must, of course, be refrigerated once it has been opened. When cold liquid formula is added to the bottle of sterile water, you may warm the bottle if you like. The baby will take it warm or cold. Personally, I prefer the powder. Most companies have perfected their products to the point where the powders dissolve easily.

The only precaution to be carefully observed occurs when a hungry baby has taken a second bottle right after the first one. Only an ounce or so may be wanted and then they're off to sleep. If *less than half an hour* has elapsed since the scoops were added to the second bottle, the remainder may be refrigerated and used for the next feeding. But if something distracts you, like the phone or the doorbell, and more than half an hour passes, discard the remainder.

The advantages of this formula technique are numerous. It is simple, flexible, and bottles with larger amounts of water can be made up so that more will be available at a time you've noticed the baby is especially hungry. This means there will be less wasted. Also, there will be no more groping out to the refrigerator in the middle of the night and standing half-asleep to warm a bottle. No more ice buckets to try to keep the bottles in your room. With this technique, you simply take your unopened bottles of water and your can of powder and mix it as you need it. When you travel, you don't need to worry about insulated bags to keep the formula from spoiling or about how you'll warm it. Just add the powder, shake, and feed. The only thing you need to remember when traveling is two pieces of tape to keep the top on the powder can to prevent a spill.

After feeding, the baby is best placed on his abdomen or right side. There has been a lot of discussion about this, but problems occur when certain details are ignored. First, the nasal passages must be clear for easy breathing. This is best done using a large or three ounce ear syringe that has a firm spring when it expands after being compressed. With the baby on its back, hold the tip of the nose up slightly so you can suction the floor of the nose. When breathing in, the air goes along the floor of the nose. When breathing out, it goes down along the spine of the nose. An infant will always struggle to get air in through the nose. Only later will the child learn it can breathe through the mouth. These days there are also electric nasal suction devices which are quite effective.

Second, when the child is placed on its abdomen, the head must be gently turned to the side to be sure the nose is not obstructed in any way by clothes or bedclothes. Almost every animal sleeps on its abdomen because the circulation is more efficient that way. The other safe position is on the right side. When stomach digestion is finished, the contents are moved to the right end of the stomach to pass through a circular muscle called the pylorus which allows passage into the first part of the small intestine for the next stage of digestion. With the baby on its right side, gravity helps the food go where it should.

Another point to know right from the start that will prevent many hours of aggravation is when the baby cries DON'T go in and pick it up immediately. Many times they'll cry once or twice, even for a few minutes, and then roll over and go back to sleep. If you run to pick it up immediately, you'll stimulate them and keep them awake when they might have slept. Then they will be a cranky, overtired baby. If it's really hunger, don't worry, the crying will continue.

Most babies have mucous which is never completely cleaned out in the nursery, even though the nurses do this many times. This mucous may occasionally cause vomiting. Though it may not seem to make sense, wait five to ten minutes and feed the baby again. It will often be retained the second time, followed by sleep. Obviously, if there is repeated vomiting, call your doctor.

Wrapping firmly, as you saw was done in the hospital, makes the baby feel secure. This is usually true for three to four weeks. After all, they've been in "close quarters" for many months.

CHAPTER 2

FEEDING — THE TRAPS THAT CAUSE TROUBLE

Babies that feed, sleep for four hours, wake and feed, and then sleep another four hours actually do exist, but they're quite rare. Most babies feed on an average of every two or three hours during the day and every three to four hours at night, but that is not intended as a pat statement. Not only do most babies have certain hungry periods during the day, but many have hungry stretches when they will take a bottle every half hour or every hour. These stretches may last two or three, even eight to ten, hours. Unless mothers realize that this may be normal for their baby, they can get very upset when they see a demand for frequent feedings. No need for frantic calls, nothing is wrong. I'll explain why.

Stop and consider for a moment, a newborn infant is growing at a very fast rate but a little stomach can hold only so much, so frequent small feedings make sense. Babies are individuals and vary as such. The rate of body growth will be different from infant to infant and nature will make each hungry according to their need. If your baby requires many feedings during the day, keep feeding. They'll probably begin to sleep through the night more quickly if you do.

The kind of baby who needs frequent feedings has caused so many young mothers who want to breast feed to give up. They feel inadequate. They think they don't have enough milk or that their milk isn't "good enough". This leads, of course, to worry and frustration, which may actually cut down on milk production. For example, a baby might take two feedings in close succession and empty both breasts. The milk hasn't built up yet. When hungry again, all that is necessary is to offer a supplemental bottle or two until the milk does come in. There is nothing over which to be worried or upset. Nothing is wrong with you, the milk, or the baby.

When a baby does get hungry, frequent feedings may be required for six to eight hours at a stretch. A small infant cannot hold a large amount of formula so concentrate the feeding by putting more powder in the same amount of water, making it richer. The proportions I usually suggest to patients are as follows:

Scoops of powder	2	$2\,1/4$	$2\,1/2$	3	$3\,1/2$
Ounces of water in bottle	4	4	4	5	6

Conversely, some babies throw up the standard 2:4 ratio and need a weaker formula for several days to a week. As they retain this and begin to get hungry, gradually increase the strength of the formula. When they can drain four ounces of the $2\,1/2$:4 concentration, they're usually big enough to hold a larger volume. Each mother can decide when her particular baby needs an increase based on the information above. Some use $2\,1/2$:4 the day after they leave the hospital, others don't make the change for three weeks. Occasionally, a very young infant will sleep for six hours after a feeding if allowed to and will awaken ravenously hungry. If this should come between 10:00 AM and 4:00 PM, you will probably be up all night feeding. Don't let a new baby sleep more than four hours from the time the last feeding was started during the day. Don't let them go over five hours at night for the first three weeks. After that, try to push the 9 to 10 PM feeding towards 11 to midnight. This will help move the 2 to 3 AM feeding nearer to 5 or 6 AM.

If you happen to have a very hungry baby who sleeps for several four hour intervals during the day and wakes frequently at night, it's perfectly alright to wake and feed every three hours during the day so the longer intervals between feedings will be at night. If the baby insists on getting days and nights mixed up, consult your doctor. A simple sedative will bring sleep at night and they'll be hungry in the morning with their schedule right side up.

Chapter 3

BREAST FEEDING

If you want to breast feed, there are a few simple things you should know. The first feedings should last only fifteen minutes. After that, the usual breast feeding time is twenty to twenty-five minutes. When the baby begins sucking, most of the milk comes out in the first five to ten minutes. During the last ten to fifteen minutes, two things are happening.

(A) The breast is drained completely and it is this complete drainage of the breast which stimulates it to produce more milk. This is why the baby should feed from one breast at one feeding and the other at the next feeding. In this way, each is drained completely and milk production is stimulated. Usually it takes three to four days for the milk to "come in". Before her breasts are filled with milk, many young mothers are worried about whether or not they'll have enough milk. The very first milk is a thick, clear, syrupy-looking liquid called colostrum. It is very concentrated and has many additional benefits to the baby in the way of extra proteins and protection against disease. A small amount is quite satisfying. Occasionally, just because the first feeding is richer than breast milk, the baby may need additional water. The only way to find out if water is necessary is to offer some. If the baby needs it, they'll take it.

Occasionally, a baby will finish a breast and still be hungry. If this happens, just offer the other breast. As mentioned at the beginning of this section, most of the milk contained in the breast will come out in the first few minutes of feeding. This should satisfy hunger but that means the second breast was not completely drained so at the next feeding, start with the breast used last so that now it will be drained completely. This will continue active milk production.

When you want to wean your baby from the breast, you do exactly the opposite. You allow feeding from both breasts each time, so that each is only partly emptied. Leaving some milk in each breast signals the body that not so much is needed. The breast glands will make less and less milk until they finally stop altogether.

(B) The second thing that happens in the last ten to fifteen minutes of feeding is the satisfying of the baby's sucking need. The newborn infant is said to be in an "oral" phase because most of their needs are satisfied or expressed by or with the mouth. Sucking is a way to satisfy a need to be active, which is different from sucking as a means of getting food when hungry. If the baby wants to be active and "let off some steam", they can't get up and run around the block. They can cry or suck. If they want to do one and can't, they'll do the other. This brings us to a consideration of pacifiers, a subject which badly needs clarification.

Chapter 4

PACIFIERS AND THUMB SUCKING

Some people are horrified at the mention of this word. Some think they should be given to all infants. The proper attitude, as with so many things, is a matter of distinguishing its *use* from its *abuse*.

In the first two months of life, an infant can't see clearly, though after one month of age it will show interest in a mobile attached to the crib or bed. Not only are they in the oral phase mentioned in the last chapter, but this sucking need increases to a peak level at about six months of age and then begins to decrease.

Just as some people have more energy and need more activity than others, babies differ too. The trick is to determine whether the baby *needs* the pacifier and to give it *only* when need is indicated. For example, after the infant has been fed and burped and is still crying, you offer the bottle again. They go at it eagerly, sucking hard, and then stop and cry. More sucking is needed but not more food. This indicates the need for the pacifier. If you give it this way, when the need slows down so will the indication.

If you give the pacifier for *your* need to keep him quiet, you'll continue giving it past the age of six months. By nine to ten months of age, there is memory and the baby has learned to get this instead of your attention. If you try to just take it away at eighteen months or two years, there'll be a terrible howl of objection.

Besides, something else has taken place. After six months, when the need normally would decrease, there is still some sucking need. When the pacifier is offered, it is taken but now the sucking is not just for food or exercise. The extra sucking has created a new, artificial need. The more the infant sucks, the more they want to suck. One day goes into another day and goes into another day and then the mother appears with a four year old and a frantic appeal, "How can I get that thing away?" If you understand what you are doing to begin with, you won't ever have the problem.

THUMB SUCKING

Some children never touch their fingers. Some take a pacifier at the proper time and never take their thumbs or fingers. Others spit out the pacifier and take their thumbs. If they are the last type, LET THEM. At this level of understanding, if you try to stop that the thought reaction is, "I like that. You are taking it away. I don't like you." But if you are the parent, they must like and depend upon you. Ergo there is conflict and confusion.

All that can be guaranteed about continually trying to pull out the thumb is that the desire for it will become even stronger. There is a classic story of an infant who had an unmarried aunt living with the family. She decided it was her sacred mission in life to stop her nephew's thumb sucking. Each time she saw him, she dutifully took it out. When he was eighteen months old, she married and left the household. He did not see her again until a family gathering when he was six years old. He had long since stopped the thumb sucking but, on entering the room and seeing her, despite the four and a half year interval, he took one look at her and put his thumb in his mouth.

Many books say a child will or should give up the thumb at two or three years. In practice, this is simply not true. Can anything be done? When is the right time to try?

The last question is the key to the answer of the first. At about the age of five, you'll find a change in children as they mature. In their play, they pretend to be grown-ups and it is an insult to have to play the baby. When the child feels this way, they can be motivated to stop. The sucking is now a habit and not a need. It needs to be replaced with a habit that says, "I don't want to do that." So calmly and casually tell this child, who now wants to be "big", "Babies suck. If you suck, you're telling me you're a baby. Do you want your milk from a bottle with a nipple?" Sometimes a five year old presented with an infant's bottle becomes so indignant they stop. Sometimes they're content to suffer the indignity of the bottle until they decide they're ready to quit. Give them the time so it's *their* decision.

Sometimes they think they'll call your bluff and say they like it. You always have more you can do though. "Babies eat baby food. Babies stay in bed all afternoon and don't go out and play with their friends." Occasionally a child may go along with all this. If they're really past the stage of development described at the beginning of this discussion, they'll draw the line at saying they like being back in diapers.

Some children only suck their thumb when they go to bed. A night light with a bottle standing near can be a simple reminder that it represents the baby they no longer want to be. All these things have one goal. When the thumb starts to the mouth, without even thinking about it, these experiences produce the thought, "I don't want that." When saying that becomes the habit, the thumb sucking stops and they can feel it's THEIR victory.

Chapter 5

SLEEP! HOW TO GET IT WHEN YOU WANT IT.

Night feedings will end any time after the baby is three weeks to three months old. Now certain other facts about the newborn can be brought out, one of the most important is whatever you do is what the baby will get used to having done. This single point is the key to many problems both now and later on in childhood.

For example, if you want a baby to go to sleep after supper and not be a problem, you must establish a regular routine, feed, burp, change if necessary, tuck in, turn out the light, close the door and leave. One extra gimmick that has been helpful is the addition to this routine of a music box toy. At three or four days of age, the baby begins to hear. If you put the music box in the crib, especially at the suppertime feeding when they're full and will probably fall asleep anyway, they'll get used to listening to this as they fall asleep. Later on, the sound of the music box will *cause* sleep. At the age of nine or ten months, you may have a tired baby who screams when removed from the family circle. If the music box has been a routine from early infancy, ten to fifteen minutes will help going off to sleep. With each pause to take a breath between cries, the tune gets through and sets off its conditioned response of sleep. This also makes traveling and visiting easier. You can go anywhere with this one little toy and as far as the baby is concerned, hearing the music means home.

If, on the other hand, you treat the baby as a new toy and go back and pick them up at the first few cries, they'll get used to this. Most importantly, they'll get overtired, which makes sleep harder to achieve. Secondly, they'll get used to too much bodily contact and come to need that. How many mothers of three or four children tell me how "good" their last baby is, but the oldest is "driving them crazy" demanding time and attention. This was the child they over-cuddled because it was a new "toy". Everyone knows about a baby's need for affection. No one has emphasized its equal need to spend some time alone. Like everything else, the time must be proportioned according to the baby's need.

It's also a good idea to have three or four toys around the crib in addition to the music box. As the child grows and is able to see more clearly, these become part of the comfortable familiarity of the sleeping routine. This prevents the dilemma of the "only one". If that certain toy is gone or the music box breaks, you don't have a major tragedy on your hands. The "rest of the team" can keep the game going.

Most babies give up a late night bottle between six weeks and three months of age. When teething starts later on or an infection or earache occurs, go in and take care and comfort but don't give a bottle. If you do, they'll start waking up for that. When comforting, don't turn on the lights in the room. Leave a light in the hall or outside somewhere, comfort them quietly, and put them back with the same sleeping routine used after supper. This is where the music box and the whole sleeping routine will help again. But if you turn on the lights and play, they'll wake up for this. After all, it's fun to have

Mommy come in, turn on the lights, and have playtime in the middle of the night.

One last word, the same one with which I began this chapter, whatever you do is what they'll get used to having done. Never put a baby into the crib to fall asleep on a bottle. Feed in your arms, in the playpen, on a mat on the floor, anywhere. The bed is for sleeping, not eating. If they fall asleep on the bottle, then this is part of the sleeping routine. That is why stopping the bottle is such a problem later on. Don't make the problem in the first place.

Another last point about position, most babies will sleep if placed on their back. Some babies, however, have very definite preferences and will sleep only on their abdomen. Don't worry about their feet turning in. If they do turn in after they've been walking for a while, that can be corrected easily. Incidentally, I purposely said, "after walking for a while". Most children turn one foot in or out when they begin to walk that makes a triangle shape with the feet. When you're unsteady, it's a lot easier to balance on three points than on two. As strength develops, most children correct this themselves.

Chapter 6

SOLIDS —WHAT, WHEN, AND WHY

It is possible to individualize the decision about when to start solid feedings. One hundred years ago, it was a radical innovation when pediatricians suggested feeding a baby solids at six months of age, babies were fed only milk until a year or more. Gradually this was moved back to three or four months. Then it became a contest. A two week old infant is not mature enough to digest food properly. It fills up the stomach and just passes through.

The system becomes mature enough to digest foods at two and a half to three months. Stomach acids are now produced in larger amounts. The drooling seen at this time is due to the maturation of the salivary glands, producing larger amounts than at birth. Some is swallowed and the rest comes out. This is *not* an indication of teething, as stated by many grandmothers. The confusion probably arose long ago because an occasional, rare baby will actually get a tooth at three months. Also when a baby does teethe later on and chew on everything they can get their hands on, that stimulates saliva and they drool.

This is why teething and drooling are associated in people's minds.

Of course, it is not always possible to wait until three to four months to start solids. As already mentioned some babies are ravenous and grow rapidly. Others eat little, but grow just as fast. Still others grow more slowly no matter how much they eat. When a baby drains six ounces of formula and is still hungry, this is the clue to start solids. Let the baby determine the time. Some need solids at five to six weeks and others not until four months. Checking weights and measurements at monthly intervals shows that each is growing normally. Normal growth rate proves the baby is getting as much nutrition as needed. I have seen babies who take nothing but formula until three to four months of age. They sleep through the night and gain and grow normally. If such a baby is given food that's not needed, it will become crampy and crabby.

As far as what foods to start are concerned, this decision should be your doctor's advice. One problem that should be stated openly here is that many pediatricians feel pressured by mothers to start solids because her girlfriend's doctor started her baby at two weeks. Let your doctor start when your baby is ready. There are far fewer serious feeding problems when the introduction of solids is determined by when YOUR baby is ready.

Chapter 7

WATER

A baby's water requirements are figured into the formula. Usually, extra water is not necessary except under special circumstances. When a newborn perspires, they lose four times as much water as an adult. During the heat of summer, when the temperature cannot be controlled, a fussy infant waking an hour or so after a feeding should be offered some water. During winter months, when room temperature can be maintained between 68 to 72 degrees Fahrenheit, this shouldn't be necessary.

This brings up another cause of family conflicts, how to dress the baby. Many people push the heat up to 80 degrees and wrap the baby to "keep them warm". But nature always tries to maintain its normal balance. When the body is too warm, perspiration begins. The evaporating sweat uses up heat. This is how the body tries to cool itself down. This "keeping warm" usually happens because someone grabs a foot, finds it cold, and thinks the baby is freezing. A baby's hands and feet are always cold because the circulation isn't well-developed yet. As long as the body is pink, they're all right.

When really cold, the skin will become blue and mottled and they will be crying. Cold feet have been the reason to make booties.

The important word on this subject is "appropriate". Dress the baby according to the temperature of the surroundings. I have seen heat exhaustion in infants who were actually swathed in woolen sweaters and blankets in July because you "have to keep a baby warm". If the thermometer hits 90 degrees, there will be perspiration in just diapers, so why put on anything else?

Occasionally, the excess perspiration is a cause of constipation. With the loss of water through the skin, the baby attempts to compensate by re-absorbing more water from the intestinal tract, leaving the contents much harder than usual. Simple constipation in an infant is often correctable by giving extra water. Enemas should never be given unless advised by your doctor.

Chapter 8

SKIN CARE

Another one of the myths that existed for centuries was that new babies had to be oiled. This was because of dry, peeling skin which we now know is just nature shedding outer layers which were surrounded by water in utero and skin better suited for the air is growing out. In some babies, this happens very slowly and only a fine peeling is noticed, if anything at all. Others look as if they had some horrible disease with the skin cracking and coming off in large flakes. This normally clears in three or four weeks. Not only is oil not necessary, but it may actually be harmful. Think how an oily film on a piece of furniture picks up dirt, the same can happen on the skin and allow infection to occur. The navel need only be touched three times a day with some alcohol or betadine. This prevents infection from developing while the cord dries up and falls off. When the navel is healed, soap can be used once a day in the bath.

A word of caution, never use perfumed soaps on a baby because their delicate skin may be sensitive to the chemicals. The best care for a new baby's skin is clear water, soap once a day as mentioned, and a little powder. Powder should never be dusted from the can, the baby is not a birthday cake. The object of using powder is to keep the skin in the folds of the fatty areas smooth and dry. Pour a little into your hand after drying the area with a towel as well as possible and smooth it into the folds. Dusting from the can creates a cloud which can be very irritating if inhaled and also allows clumps of powder to remain in the folds.

Care of the head is simple. Hair is a naturally oily area. It should not be shampooed daily or the natural oil will be removed. On shampoo days, twice a week, if you feel that your baby's head is very dry, rub in a little oil. You may find yourself using this twice a week or not at all. Cradle cap occurs when the flaky skin of the scalp is not removed. Do not be afraid to wash over the "soft spot". You are not near the baby's brain, which is covered with thick, canvas-like protecting membranes over a layer of fluid. A washcloth or soft brush will clean this area nicely.

The breast swelling you see in both male and female infants is due to the effect of all the hormones that were active in your body during pregnancy, some of which passed over to the baby and cause this. Occasionally, you may even see a drop of milk ooze from a nipple. NEVER, NEVER squeeze or press the breasts, that may cause an abscess. Leave them alone. The effect will be gone after a month or so.

Infant girls may have a vaginal discharge and on the third or fourth day you may even see a slight bloody discharge. This is called physiologic menstruation and is perfectly normal. It is also from those transferred hormones. Just wash with clear water. It will usually be gone in a day or two.

Another problem to check for, which can be simply and easily corrected in the female infant and which can prevent a problem later on is to see if there is labial fusion. Occasionally, I would find that the infant labia were stuck together. Just separating them with a thumb on each side will separate them easily. Sometimes a tiny bit of bleeding may be seen, putting some Vaseline on each side will prevent them from sticking together again. If this is not discovered and corrected in the infant, skin will grow there and the vaginal opening may be partially or even completely covered. At maturity, this can interfere with normal menstrual flow and sexual relations.

I had one mother who told me of trouble she and her husband had during their first month of marriage. She was a virgin but had been able to use a tampon during menstruation. They were unable to achieve normal sexual congress. He thought she was deliberately giving him a hard time and was understandably angry. She couldn't understand what was wrong. It took a month before they realized a gynecologist should be consulted. Skin was partially covering the vaginal opening allowing only enough access for a tampon. She had to have surgical separation of the fused labia. Examination and correction in infancy could have prevented that. This is also why it is advisable for teenage girls to begin seeing a gynecologist. I sent my daughters to start seeing a gynecologist when they were sixteen.

Chapter 9

ELIMINATION

Normally, the number of movements may vary between one and eight per day. Some babies soil a diaper after each feeding. Others do so once a day. *Frequency* of movement does NOT constitute diarrhea. This is determined by the character of the movement. One completely liquid, watery stool is diarrhea. Eight normal formed movements are NOT.

Color may vary from light yellow to gray-green to dark brown. The green stools everyone is warned about are green, watery stools. Many babies between the ages of two to six weeks normally pass gray-green formed stools. This is not due to the introduction of solids. I have seen this in many infants, including my own, who were on nothing but formula.

Consistency will vary too, from soft or seedy to firm "pebbles". If it appears regularly without undue trouble, don't worry. Often a young infant will pass a formed stool with a ring of stained water around it. As long as there is form to the major portion, it is not diarrhea. If the entire stool is liquid, call your doctor.

Chapter 10

SNEEZES, STUFFINESS AND HICCUPS

Just a brief note on these in passing, the lining of the nose produces a normal amount of mucous for lubrication. The small opening of the infant nostril can become blocked by this normal production. Nature has provided the sneeze reflex to keep the nasal passages clear. A series of sneezes several times a day is quite common.

The best way to clear the baby's nose is with a three ounce size ear syringe. There are nasal aspirators on the market but the bulb is usually too small to create effective suction. Even the one and two ounce ear syringes are too small. I've found the three ounce size works best. Be sure to get a bulb that has a good "spring" or resiliency so that it will expand quickly. Avoid one that is soft and expands slowly. Just compressing it and putting the tip into the baby's nostril, which may admit the tip about an eighth of an inch before it's a snug fit, and then releasing the bulb quickly so it can expand and pull out any nasal mucous which is causing stuffiness will give immediate relief.

Usually a tissue or paper towel can be used on to which you can empty the contents of the bulb and then repeat the suctioning. This can be continued five, ten, fifteen times, as many as necessary to get clear breathing. If you see a streak of blood, stop suctioning. Occasionally a small blood vessel in the lining will break. Leave it alone. It will heal quickly by itself. If bleeding continues, twist a bit of cotton and insert it into the nostril, but in eighteen years I've never heard of this being needed.

With some newborn infants, you may find it necessary to suction once or twice a day until, at two or three months of age, the nasal passages are a little bigger and the small amount of mucous normally produced is no longer enough to cause them to be stuffy. If a cold develops, using the ear syringe this way makes it possible for you to give quick relief until you call for specific medical advice. Nothing is more frustrating than to listen to a baby sniffle during the night and not be able to help. This technique will at least help you to provide temporary relief. As mentioned in Chapter 1, there are also electric nasal suction devices.

Some babies never get hiccups and some do constantly. If you ignore them, they'll disappear in twenty to thirty minutes. All the remedies that have been dreamed up to "treat" them are really to keep you occupied until all is well again.

Chapter 11

OUTDOORS AND INDOORS

Babies will usually do better if they get some fresh air each day, provided you are not in an area with smog or pollution. In the summer, going outdoors can start at two weeks but be sure their face and eyes are protected. Remember the sun moves during the day and even if it is not directly on their face when first out, be sure it does not get into the eyes after a while.

As was mentioned in Chapter 7, clothing should be appropriate for the actual conditions. In colder months, wait for three or four weeks to start. A simple guide you can use is this.

>At 8 lbs, not below 60 degrees F
>At 10 lbs, not below 50 degrees F

Exposure to the sun must be done carefully because newborn skin is very delicate. Start with a minute or two once a day on the chest and abdomen. Gradually increase this until you reach half an hour. In bad weather, a substitute might be to dress the baby for outdoors but use a room with the window open and the door closed. Babies who get fresh air each day, even for short periods, seem to have better appetites and do well.

According to Dr. Michael Holick of Boston University, an international authority on vitamin D, infant skin does make vitamin D in response to sunlight. Its role in helping the absorption of calcium is critical for growth, not only for the development of bones and teeth but also for nerve and muscle development and function. Dr. Holick says fifteen to thirty minutes a day of natural sun will produce the necessary amount of vitamin D for a growing child if it is mid-morning or mid- to late afternoon sun and the damaging 10:00 AM to 2:00 PM noonday rays will be avoided.

Though babies get vitamin drops with D, scientific experience has taught that there may be things happening in normal physiologic processes of which we are still unaware. This is why it is best to attempt a balance between enough sunlight to create vitamin D normally and preventing excessive exposure to avoid sun damage.

Chapter 12

TOILET TRAINING OR, BETTER STILL, "LEARNING CONTROL"

The trouble with this expression is that the word "training" is unconsciously understood as it would be with an adult as a responsibility of one person to get an idea across to another about performing a certain task. But now we're concerned with a developing child, not an adult. This can be understood more clearly by a simple explanation of general development and maturation.

When a baby is born, most of the nerve cells in the brain still have a lot of growing to do. The cells that will help the child move have to extend part of themselves out like a long cable to the parts they will control. At birth, those "cables" are very short. A baby's movements at birth are completely random, completely by chance. A hand, for example, may wind up in the mouth just by chance. Then, while sucking on it, the hand will move away and they'll cry. They don't yet have the control to put it back where they want it. The lengthening part of the nerve cells grows down from the brain. As they get to the neck muscles, the head can be picked up more securely. It doesn't wobble as much as it did at first.

At three months or so, the shoulders and arms are reached and now the hands can be put where they want them to go. This is when a playpen can be used. They can reach for and bat their hands at a crib gym or any simple object you string in front of them. They can't grab or hold it yet. That will come when the nerves get to the hands and fingers. As the nerves grow down to the trunk, hips, and thighs, the ability to roll over, sit up, and crawl will come, when nerves grow to the legs and feet, standing and walking.

Biologically speaking, we have learned to get around standing on our hind legs. Though that may seem odd, the point is that the very *last* muscles to get the nerves, and therefore to be controlled, are those at the tail end, the muscles which control bowel and bladder functions.

Our individual time clocks make each action happen at a certain time, a little different for each of us. I have seen children walk at eight or nine months and others not until they were over two years old. Some children can control bowel and bladder action at eighteen months and some not until after three years. Suppose a particular child were going to walk at eighteen months of age. When he was only fifteen months, you wouldn't dream of suddenly deciding, "I'm going to walk train you now." What would you think of someone who tried to force a child to stand up and walk when his body was not yet ready?

Trying to "train" a child at a time when *you* think they should be ready is doing the same thing. The mother who thinks she must get this done by a certain time and then finds she can't will be frustrated and unnecessarily so. She thinks she's not doing a good job as a mother.

NONSENSE!

When your child shows they can pull themselves up to stand and then tries a few steps, getting ready to walk, you help them. They're learning by themselves what their body can do. You just offer help at the right time, but you don't *teach them* to walk. You can't. You instinctively understand that. They've tried, for example, taking identical twins and giving one of them special exercises and leg training to see if that one would walk sooner. I'm sure you're not surprised to learn they walked at the same time. When the nerves have grown down to supply the muscles, then those muscles can perform their intended function. When your child doesn't soil repeatedly and seems to stay clean and dry for longer periods, you can begin putting them on a seat on the toilet.

Try to catch them at the right time. It's just a matter of chance the first time they actually do something on the toilet. When you applaud and praise this coincidence, they quickly make the association of doing this and getting your approval. NEVER make the mistake of thinking, "I'll praise when this is done and scold when there's soiling." They never in their little lives have *been* completely trained. If you do this, their experience is suddenly being spanked or scolded for something they've always done and that's very confusing. What they're starting to learn is very complicated, to get the sensation of needing to eliminate, control it, remember to communicate to you somehow that it's time to go, and then continue to control until helped to the proper place. This is a significant set of associations for a little one to accomplish.

One very important thing to know is that, before being completely trained, they'll often come and tell you AFTER their pants are soiled. This happens *just before* complete control develops. They've understood that you want something of them in relation to this function and they're trying to do what you want. Always give praise for them having came and told you. As the nerves continue to grow and mature, they become aware of the sensation *before* soiling and, remembering approval, now come at that time. Now control of these muscles and functions has been learned along with when and where.

The next time some older woman looks down her nose at you and says, "What? Haven't you trained your child yet?" tell her to go jump in the lake.

Chapter 13

SAFETY POINTS AND SOME COMMENTS ON "FRIENDLY ADVICE"

As we just discussed, a very young baby's arms flail about in completely random movements. There is no control. One of the most tragic things that can happen to a family is having the baby everyone has waited for, and is prepared to love, do permanent damage to a parent's eye. Their nails grow quickly and their arms move rapidly. Whenever your face is within reach of those hands, have your eyes half closed and be ready to close them instantly if a hand moves near them. A quick flick of a baby's nail can take a chunk out of an adult's eye. Depending upon where in the eye this happens, it may cause serious and permanent damage. Being aware of this danger can prevent a lot of heartache. You can buy special blunt baby scissors to keep the nails cut short. This also prevents them from scratching themselves.

Don't get used to the baby not being able to move. Always strap them in to protect from falling off a table or bassinet. With the random movements of arms and legs, occasionally a foot may catch the surface on which they're lying in a particular way and stretching a leg can cause a flip over. Many people misinterpret this as a baby turning over at one and a half to two months of age. The important thing is to prevent harm.

Just another cautionary word on a familiar subject, never let an infant get hold of objects small enough to get into the mouth. Older siblings must be cautioned against giving the baby beads or the like.

Baseball has really been replaced as the American national pastime. The national pastime now is telling *other* people how to bring up *their* children. Young parents with a first baby are always choice targets. Well-meaning friends and relatives will not only suggest things, they'll state them with a great tone of authority. Usually, they are wrong. At times, there is a grain of truth or a very specific point lurking under the mass of exaggeration but it is often distorted. If what you hear worries and upsets you, check with your doctor, even if it seems like a small thing. This is better than stewing over it for days, which will do nobody any good.

Most new mothers get some kind of help, either from family or a nurse. This help should consist of doing housework and cooking. She should take care of her baby *herself* to get the feel of it. If her help takes care of the infant then when they leave, she will findsherself with all her routine work and she's not yet used to the baby. Obviously, she has not really been helped. An experienced mother, on the other hand, is more likely to want someone to handle the infant.

Chapter 14

SOME GENERAL POINTS ABOUT SICKNESS AND WHAT YOU SHOULD KNOW ABOUT FEVER

Fever is not a "must" to indicate sickness. Much more valid is a change in the general pattern of the baby's behavior and/or eating. All of us in Pediatrics have a healthy respect for the seemingly vague statement, "Doctor, I don't know what's wrong but this is just not my baby."

A first infection often appears right after a Christening or a family affair. This is the time when parents have a perfect right to be firm. Let the family call you names. Nothing is worse for a new infant than fifty people picking them up and breathing and coughing all over them. No matter how close a relative may be, they can still be a source of infection.

Fever is a defense against invading germs. It develops because the body shuts down the ways it loses heat, keeping more heat inside. What we usually call dry skin has a certain amount of moisture in it. You can tell the difference when you feel the hot, dry skin of someone with fever. The water usually in the skin evaporates slowly and uses up some heat, since it requires heat to change water to water vapor. When the water is kept from getting out of the skin because the sweat glands are shut down then heat is kept in the body. Hands and feet are usually cold because circulation is slowed down in these areas. The reason for this is that heat is lost more quickly and easily from a point than from a flat, thick, or round surface. This is why people with fever often have cold hands and feet. Since by definition fever means "too much heat," you never need to be afraid of "chilling" anyone with fever. If you put extra clothes and blankets on a feverish patient, you are *adding* to what the body is doing naturally. If a child has fever of 102 and you wrap them in extra blankets, you can push that to 104.

When a patient has chills and fever, something else is happening due to the infection. That patient feels cold even with a fever of 105. In this case, of course, you must cover up. The sweating causes heat loss and often can relieve the chills too, BUT it has no effect on the cause of the illness. It does nothing to the germ that started it. If your doctor has instructed you to give medicine to reduce the fever, it usually wears off in about four hours. That's why you're asked to check the temperature every four hours to tell what the fever really is. Two hours after giving the medicine, the temperature may be down to 100 or 101, but after four hours you will know the true level of the fever.

One word of caution, feeling a child's forehead can be very deceiving. The only way to actually know about fever is to take the temperature rectally! Sick, upset, or excited children occasionally bite a thermometer that is in their mouth and then you've got additional problems.

Body temperature does not stay at 98.6 all the time. Normally, it goes down a degree or two when we sleep. That's why it may be 96.5 or 97 first thing in the morning. As we move through the day, it often goes to 99.6 or 99.8. Especially in an active child, anything under 100 rectally is really not a fever. This is also why, when there is illness, their temperature may be normal in the morning and a fever comes later in the day. Fever anytime during a twenty-four hour period is considered a "fever day". This is why temperature remaining under 100 for forty-eight hours consecutively indicates the end of the sickness. As mentioned at the beginning of this chapter, fever is not the end all and be all. Some children and adults can be quite sick without fever. When a doctor considers an ill patient, many things are taken into account. Fever is only one of them.

One last important point about illness generally, if an antibiotic is prescribed, you should understand it takes time to act. Some antibiotics have an effect in twenty-four to thirty-six hours and some not for forty-eight hours. Before these medications were available, the natural course of a sore throat or bronchitis was ten days to three weeks. That's why, when they were first available during and just after World War II, a response in two or three days was spectacular. Don't expect that your child will be cured after two doses.

Chapter 15

HOW TO GIVE NOSE DROPS TO TREAT NASAL PROBLEMS AND TO RELIEVE EARACHE.

Most people are used to getting a terrible fight from a child when the subject of nose drops comes up. This is because they were given incorrectly the first time they were used. If you just drop the liquid into the center of the nostril, it falls directly to the back of the nose, burns that area, and the child is not about to let you do *that* again. Even worse, it's ineffective.

When there is an infection, the lining or wall of each nostril is inflamed and swollen. *This* is where you want the drops. Put the tip of the dropper into the nostril and tilt it slightly so you deposit the drops on the lining of each nostril. Now it will spread out over the wall and run down inside gradually. This prevents the burning from the concentrated drop hitting that back wall. More importantly, the medicine has a chance to act where it's needed.

Nose drops used properly this way are also the fastest way to relieve the severe pain of an earache. The middle ear and the back of the nose are connected by a small tube called the

Eustachian tube. When infection gets back into the nose and spreads out through this tube to the middle ear, the inflammation and swelling cause the inner end of this tube to become swollen shut. As the infected area produces mucous and pus, it's now trapped under pressure in a closed space. The eardrum slowly bulges to compensate for the pressure so the pain eases somewhat. When pressure builds again, pain recurs. Pain and then easing is the natural course of an ear infection. Sometimes the pressure in the middle ear will rise too fast for the eardrum to accommodate, then there will be relief of pain when the eardrum bursts. NEVER be fooled when a child says, "It doesn't hurt anymore". The relief is only temporary. The complaint of earache means something is going on and it should have immediate medical attention.

If the right ear hurts, for example, lay the child flat on their back and put four or five nose drops into the right nostril, depositing them on the lining of the side wall as mentioned previously. Keep them lying flat for five minutes so the drops can run back to shrink down the swelling around the inner end of the Eustachian tube and open it up. Then, after five minutes, roll the head to the opposite side so they're lying on their left cheek. With the right ear up, the fluid under pressure can run down the tube to the back of the nose. Try to keep this position for about five minutes. If this doesn't relieve the earache, repeat it every fifteen to twenty minutes until you *do* get relief. The most I've ever seen needed is a third time. Usually the second will do the trick. Obviously, if the left ear hurts, put the drops in the left nostril and follow the above instructions, turning onto the right cheek after five minutes.

If both ears are painful, put the drops as directed into both nostrils and just keep the child flat for five minutes then allow them to get up. Normal movements will drain both ears. You can't turn to either side in this case because what will improve one will make the other worse.

These simple instructions about properly using nose drops

enable parents to do something quickly at home to give their crying child relief from ear pain or relieve restlessness from stuffiness and obstructed breathing. If the nose is suctioned first with the ear syringe (as described in chapter 10), the nose drops will be even more effective.

Most nose drops have a decongesting, shrinking agent. Instructions vary with different ones from use every three to four hours to those lasting twelve to twenty-four hours. No matter what the instructions for regular use when relieving an earache, use them every fifteen to twenty minutes as described until the child's pain is gone.

But don't be fooled by the absence of pain, YOU MUST CALL THE DOCTOR ABOUT THE EARACHE.

Chapter 16

VOMITING AND DIARRHEA – HOW TO CONTROL MOST CASES USING CLEAR LIQUIDS AND CAREFUL FEEDING

Basically, the principles are the same for both conditions in children and adults, with one obvious exception, when there is diarrhea, the liquids *which are permitted* can be taken freely. With vomiting, they must be taken cautiously, offering small amounts at five to ten minute intervals.

1.) ALL foods must be stopped especially NO MILK, NO SOUP, and NO FRUIT JUICE. Fatty foods are very irritating. Even skim milk and clear broth have enough fat left in them to set off the vomiting and diarrhea again. The normal milk sugar can be irritating. Fruits have substances which are naturally irritating to the intestinal tract, which is why they are natural laxatives. This is the last thing you want.

Many of the older generation rush to give a sick person soup, especially barley soup, and juices. This is because, when the importance of fluids in illness began to be appreciated, any tasty fluid preparations were suggested as a means of getting the patient to take liquids. Most people like barley soup and *that's* why doctors often suggested it. Then people got the mistaken notion that there was something curative about the barley. It was the liquid that was important. With these symptoms in the intestinal tract, the soup is contra-indicated.

The only liquids permitted for the patient with vomiting and/or diarrhea from infection or irritation are weak tea (with no more than a teaspoon of sugar to 8 oz. of weak tea if it is refused plain), ginger ale, and salted water using one half teaspoon of salt to 8 oz. of water. With diarrhea, plain water is also allowed. When vomiting, plain water is not well tolerated and will probably come up. ANY of the above liquids should not be given to a vomiting patient until there has been no vomiting for at least one and a half to two hours. Then offer very small amounts at a time for example a teaspoonful every five minutes if necessary. A baby can be given fluids by the dropper if the stomach is very sensitive or allowed to suck only half an ounce at a time from the bottle.

Clear liquids should be continued until there has been no vomiting or diarrhea *for twenty-four hours.* I emphasize this point because so many times when this has not worked, mothers have said, "I gave the tea and ginger ale for twenty-four hours and then started other foods." These liquids should be given until *there has been no vomiting or diarrhea* for twenty-four hours. That's when the next step can be introduced.

2.) Dry toast with no butter, dry water crackers, bananas, and boiled mashed carrots. Because bananas are often recommended to patients with diarrhea, people mistakenly think they are constipating. It is due to the fact that the sugar in bananas is simple sugar – dextrose – and doesn't have to be broken down (i.e., digested) to be absorbed. Thus, it is non-irritating. Carrots have a naturally soothing and coating property which lines the intestinal tract and helps to quiet the increased activity causing the diarrhea.

When these few simple foods, still with the clear liquids, have been tolerated for another twenty-four hours, with no recurrence of the vomiting or diarrhea, then the next stage of the diet can be offered.

> 3.) Skim milk, cereals (oatmeal or cold cereals which are not sugary or flavored), applesauce, boiled rice, jello, custards, potatoes (no butter or other flavoring), and cottage cheese.

When these foods have been tolerated for another twenty-four hours with no symptoms, then a regular diet may be resumed, leaving heavy, fatty foods like soups, meats, and eggs as the last to be re-introduced.

Chapter 17

AVOIDING EATING PROBLEMS IN CHILDREN

As with any other subject, the first need to fill is information. Proper information will relieve parental guilt. Metabolic rates (i.e., how fast a baby grows) change during the stages of infancy and childhood. Proper information about these changes is critical to understanding, solving, and preventing eating problems, especially their development into interpersonal power plays.

The newborn infant grows rapidly. Birth weight doubles in three to four months. By one year, this rate slacks off. The average eighteen month old does not eat as much as a six month old. Not knowing this, a mother will worry needlessly. At two years of age, insulating baby fat is lost as the developing nervous system becomes better at regulating body temperature and metabolic rate slows considerably.

The reality and importance of this was learned after World War II and the starvation conditions that existed, even outside the concentration camps. Pediatricians examining children in late 1945 and 1946 were amazed to find normal growth in the two to six year olds. The growth spurt between six and nine and, of course, adolescence were understandably affected.

Not knowing that these changes are normal causes maternal distress. "I'm not getting good nutrition into my child. I'm an irresponsible parent." That's how the problem starts, trying to force food into a child who's not hungry. How would you feel if someone were trying to force you to eat and you didn't want to?

YOUR CHILD IS NOT GOING TO STARVE.

Let me tell you about an actual experience with one of my patients to make the point. I'd just finished an annual exam on a three year old boy. As his mother was leaving, she turned back and said, "I'm having a terrible time getting him to eat. Can you suggest anything?"

I reviewed the normal changes in nutritional need and then, reassuring her he would not starve, I advised her not to pressure him if he didn't want to eat and just to give him water, NOT MILK. She was surprised by that. We made another appointment for a month to follow up on this.

Her story at the next visit was as follows:

> The next morning, I got him dressed but he didn't want breakfast. I gave him just the water and let him go and play. At noon, he didn't want lunch. Again, I gave him just water and he went to play with his toys. He didn't want dinner either. He took some water. I gave him his bath, read him a story, and put him to bed.
>
> On the second morning, he still didn't want breakfast but took some water and went to play. At lunch on that second day, I decided not to say anything but put a sandwich, a glass of milk, and a piece of fruit on the table. He came in, gobbled it up, and I haven't had a problem with him since.

Question: When does food taste best?
Answer: When you're hungry.
Explanation: She'd given him a chance to enjoy his food. The opportunity to enjoy food is missing when food is forced on someone who's not hungry. What about choices? It's perfectly acceptable to insist on a "taste". Some children will refuse a food without tasting when food has become part of a power play. If they don't want something, that's okay. But, "That's what we're having for dinner. You don't have to eat it if you don't want it." The biggest mistake is making "something special" just so the child will eat. This creates the power play. It is always a set-up for trouble when power is in the hands of someone immature with inadequate experience on which to base a judgment. Even worse than that, making "something special" sends a destructive subconscious message to the child. "You're unable to eat what everyone else can because you're inadequate." It's the same principle as a mother tying the shoelaces of an eight year old. The unconscious message is, "I'm doing this because I don't think you're able to do it yourself." Believe me! These subconscious messages are read and understood loud and clear.

Since whatever you eat when you're hungry will taste good, the most nutritionally destructive thing an adult can do is offer a hungry child a sweet snack - a cookie, a lollipop, or some candy. One of my patient's mothers had been heavy as a child. She'd worked very hard getting to a normal weight. Her children, she'd determined, were not going to have that problem. As toddlers, if they wanted a snack it would be fruit, cheese, or, when they had their molars and could chew well, raw vegetables like string beans with the ends cut off, a piece of celery spread with cream cheese, a piece of tomato, a slice of block cheese on an unsalted water biscuit, a slice of a green or red pepper or cucumber, etc. As they began to be invited to friend's birthday parties, she told them they were free to eat the ice cream, cake, and candy but found they had no taste for those things. When they were older, they did eat these things, but never to excess and they were never overweight.

To prevent or solve any problem, the key is always getting as much valid information as possible and to continue getting and checking information from different sources so you can practice your freedom to keep improving.

Chapter 18

SOME POINTS ABOUT GROWTH AND DEVELOPMENT

Growth in height and weight does not occur steadily. A baby, and later a child, grows in spurts and plateaus. This is true not only for height and weight but for the development of learning both mentally and physically.

Some babies do not gain from one month's visit to the next then they increase strikingly. I've seen babies who didn't grow on three successive monthly visits and then shot up on the next. Never compare your baby's size to a friend's baby. When you see one person who is five foot five and another who is six foot one you don't wonder why they're not the same size. Why expect babies to grow alike?

At the end of the first year, somewhere between nine and thirteen months of age, the rate of growth slows markedly. The baby's appetite also falls off, as mentioned in the previous chapter. Sometimes this is a sudden, drastic decrease, but sometimes it's gradual or not even noticeable. Knowing this will happen will prevent worry when it does. Another thing which can interfere with eating at the end of the first year is teething.

The age-old question always returns: Does teething cause fever? Probably not, but many babies seem to have low-grade fever (101 – 101.5) for several days and then this clears when the tooth comes through. This may be a short viral illness coincidental with the tooth's appearance. Anyone who is strongly convinced it's the tooth will not be swayed by what I've said. However, one point is important. If the temperature goes over 102, better check on it. It's probably not the tooth.

Later on, walking, talking, and learning new skills will develop the same way. If you find yourself saying, "Nothing new seems to have been learned in a long time," two weeks later you'll be amazed at what can suddenly be done or understood.

Chapter 19

DISCIPLINE

Disciplining a child is the only real way you can let them know you love and care for them. Setting rules and limits conveys the fact that you've taken on the responsibility to decide what they need and then to enforce that decision. After the feeding, snuggling, and caring for their needs during infancy, proper discipline is the most significant way you can show you really care about their welfare. I'll explain what I mean about "proper" discipline in more detail later on.

So many parents ask me, "How do you know when to be strict with a child and when do you start?" A useful guide for deciding when to be strict is when the situation concerns the child's safety. Decide to be dramatic and emphatic when the result may be traumatic.

You can't begin this much before two to two and a half years of age and the situation must be simple and clear-cut enough for the child to grasp it. If the child picks up a knife or scissors or goes to touch something hot, exaggerate your voice and give it a fierce tone that will attract their attention.

If the tone change is not obeyed — and some children won't – follow it up with action. Hold their arm firmly and take away the dangerous tool. Then they'll realize that this tone in your voice means business. You have to know your child, of course. Some will obey and some will not. But a hug combined with firm words that this is not to be done will convey that this is "something different".

IMPORTANT: Don't expect a two or three-year-old to remember and conform the next time. They have not yet developed the ability to have self-control. That doesn't come until five or six.

Some are naturally iron-willed and persistent, so you have to be more so. If they know this tone has special meaning then, when a little older and possibly in a dangerous situation like climbing or walking somewhere where there's a chance of trauma, your voice can stop and protect them. If they're used to ignoring you, the results could be tragic.

As I just mentioned, before the age of five or six, the child does not have the ability to control themselves. Just as they could not walk when the nervous system was not mature enough, they can't control impulses to investigate their surroundings – to touch, to bite, to taste, to push or pull, or to hit. You, the parent, have to be that control. The most frustrating part of early years is feeling you're a failure because they keep doing what you tell them not to do. Knowing they're unable to control their behavior helps you understand you're *not* a failure, just as you would have been unable to get them to walk before they were ready. You are providing the control the immature nervous system cannot yet accomplish.

At five or six, the child takes into themselves whatever the parent's attitudes have been. That is why the general rule is if you don't discipline a child during the first five years of life it will be harder for them later to discipline themselves. Self-discipline is the key to "I must do this," "I must not do that," or "I must finish this homework assignment on time." This is what creates the inner strength that leads to success later in life. Your continuing to be the control gives the gift of how to survive, which is the basic role of any parent. This enables, "I have to stand the pain of this shot because I will be better afterwards" or "Fun will have to wait until I get the job done."

The other big gift is learning that they CAN do things if they have to, which leads to less fear and more confidence in themselves. Such as, "that shot hurt but I was able to stand the pain". Life will have many unpleasant things in store but they won't be "thrown" if they know they CAN survive. They will have the supreme gift of being able to depend upon themselves. This is the kind of person who can come across a piece of work ten years later and be able to say, "I know that was well done because *I* did it." The internal comfort provided by knowledge of self-worth starts with a parent caring enough to discipline and control the child before they can do it themselves.

There are other results of your discipline. When in school there are safety classes, the connection is suddenly made that your "don't touch that" and "keep away from there" were showing your concern for their well-being. This really shows your love and reinforces a sense of self-worth. Showing how to protect them from danger is part of the basic parental role of teaching survival.

Words and actions also have implied meanings. Though these are understood subconsciously they are, nevertheless, understood very clearly. When you make a child do or learn something that's, ultimately, for their safety or welfare — as in setting a limit — despite the grumbling objection, they understand you care about them. This includes social behavior. If you think you're being kind by reversing a decision and saying, "Well okay, you don't have to," the unconscious message received is you really didn't care what they did. It means you're more interested in having the child *like you* than in recognizing a *need for guidance*. It may also lead to more unruly behavior which is their way of saying, "please care enough to take a stand." They'll also sense they can't come to this parent for help. The corollary to this, "I don't have to if I don't want to" is not the path to success.

At the beginning of this discussion, I mentioned "proper" discipline. Improper discipline is sending the message, "You do it this way because I want *my children* to do this." This implies no recognition of the child's individuality but that they are only an extension of the parent. You are MY child as differentiated from my CHILD. They insist on a child behaving a certain way because of how it makes *them* look.

Proper discipline includes cuddling, playing, and *telling* the child that they're loved. One key to a child's thought processes is the word "literal". Exactly what you say is exactly what you mean. You can say to a child, "I want you to do this (or not do that) because I love you and want what's best for you." Underneath the outward grumbling at the restriction, they'll be pleased and comforted. When a child tells friends, "I have to do this because my folks are really strict," the message they're giving to those friends is that you really care about them.

Don't expect that either you or your children will have all success or all happiness. Everyone knows life has ups and downs, happiness and sorrow. The goal of good parenting is helping children learn how to handle the hurdles.

www.ingramcontent.com/pod-product-compliance
Lightning Source LLC
Chambersburg PA
CBHW061517180526
45171CB00001B/217